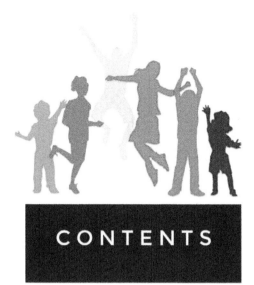

CONTENTS

- ❖ **PERSONALIZATION PAGE**
- ❖ **PARENT(S) / GUARDIANS INFORMATION**
- ❖ **EXTENDED MEDICAL INFORMATION**
- ❖ **FAMILY MEDICAL HISTORY**
- ❖ **INSURANCE DETAILS**
- ❖ **IMMUNIZATION RECORD**
- ❖ **TREATMENT HISTORY- MEDICATION**
- ❖ **SYMPTOM TRACKER**
- ❖ **TREATMENT HISTORY- VISITS**
- ❖ **GROWTH LOG**
- ❖ **WEIGHT LOG**
- ❖ **TEETH CHARTS**
- ❖ **NOTES PAGES**

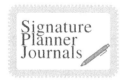

www.signatureplannerjournals.com
www.signatureplannerjournals.co.uk

THIS BOOK BELONGS TO

NAME		Gender	
D.O.B		Place Of Birth	
BIRTH WEIGHT		Birth Length	
ADDRESS			

Eye Color		Skin Color		
Blood Group		Organ Donor?	Yes	No
Medical Conditions				
Allergies				

EMERGENCY CONTACT 1

NAME	
RELATIONSHIP	
CONTACT NUMBER	
ADDRESS	
NOTES	

EMERGENCY CONTACT 2

NAME	
RELATIONSHIP	
CONTACT NUMBER	
ADDRESS	
NOTES	

PARENTS/ GUARDIANS

NAME		Gender	
D.O.B	Place Of Birth		
ADDRESS			
BLOOD GROUP		Organ Donor?	Yes	No
MEDICAL CONDITIONS			
ALLERGIES			

NAME		Gender	
D.O.B	Place Of Birth		
ADDRESS			
BLOOD GROUP		Organ Donor?	Yes	No
MEDICAL CONDITIONS			
ALLERGIES			

NOTES

EXTENDED MEDICAL INFORMATION

EXTENDED MEDICAL INFORMATION

FAMILY MEDICAL HISTORY

MOTHER / MATERNAL GRANDPARENTS	YES	NO	NOTES
High Blood Pressure			
Stroke			
High Cholesterol			
Diabetes			
Glaucoma			
Epilepsy			
Asthma			
Obesity			
Allergies			
Cancer (type)			
Hearing Loss			
Alcohol Misuse			
Drug Misuse			
Kidney Problems			

FATHER / PATERNAL GRANDPARENTS	YES	NO	NOTES
High Blood Pressure			
Stroke			
High Cholesterol			
Diabetes			
Glaucoma			
Epilepsy			
Asthma			
Obesity			
Allergies			
Cancer (type)			
Hearing Loss			
Alcohol Misuse			
Drug Misuse			
Kidney Problems			

INSURANCE DETAILS

COMPANY	
POLICY DETAILS	
COVER DETAILS	
ADDRESS	
CONTACT NO.	
EMAIL	
WEBSITE	

HEALTH CARE DETAILS

PEDIATRICIAN DETAILS	
NAME:	
ADDRESS:	
PHONE NUMBER:	

DENTIST	
NAME:	
ADDRESS:	
PHONE NUMBER:	

SPECIALIST	
NAME:	
DETAILS:	
ADDRESS:	
PHONE NUMBER:	

COMPANY	
POLICY DETAILS	
COVER DETAILS	
ADDRESS	
CONTACT NO.	
EMAIL	
WEBSITE	

HEALTH CARE DETAILS

PEDIATRICIAN DETAILS	
NAME:	
ADDRESS:	
PHONE NUMBER:	

DENTIST	
NAME:	
ADDRESS:	
PHONE NUMBER:	

SPECIALIST	
NAME:	
DETAIL:	
ADDRESS:	
PHONE NUMBER:	

IMMUNIZATION RECORD

Vaccine:

Date administered:

Next Dose date:

Administered by:

Vaccine:

Date administered:

Next Dose date:

Administered by:

Vaccine:

Date administered:

Next Dose date:

Administered by:

Vaccine:

Date administered:

Next Dose date:

Administered by:

Vaccine:

Date administered:

Next Dose date:

Administered by:

Vaccine:

Date administered:

Next Dose date:

Administered by:

Vaccine:

Date administered:

Next Dose date:

Administered by:

Vaccine:

Date administered:

Next Dose date:

Administered by:

Vaccine:

Date administered:

Next Dose date:

Administered by:

Vaccine:

Date administered:

Next Dose date:

Administered by:

Vaccine:

Date administered:

Next Dose date:

Administered by:

Vaccine:

Date administered:

Next Dose date:

Administered by:

IMMUNIZATION RECORD

Vaccine:

Date administered:

Next Dose date:

Administered by:

Vaccine:

Date administered:

Next Dose date:

Administered by:

Vaccine:

Date administered:

Next Dose date:

Administered by:

Vaccine:

Date administered:

Next Dose date:

Administered by:

Vaccine:

Date administered:

Next Dose date:

Administered by:

Vaccine:

Date administered:

Next Dose date:

Administered by:

IMMUNIZATION RECORD

Vaccine:

Date administered:

Next Dose date:

Administered by:

Vaccine:

Date administered:

Next Dose date:

Administered by:

Vaccine:

Date administered:

Next Dose date:

Administered by:

Vaccine:

Date administered:

Next Dose date:

Administered by:

Vaccine:

Date administered:

Next Dose date:

Administered by:

Vaccine:

Date administered:

Next Dose date:

Administered by:

IMMUNIZATION RECORD

Vaccine:

Date administered:

Next Dose date:

Administered by:

Vaccine:

Date administered:

Next Dose date:

Administered by:

Vaccine:

Date administered:

Next Dose date:

Administered by:

Vaccine:

Date administered:

Next Dose date:

Administered by:

Vaccine:

Date administered:

Next Dose date:

Administered by:

Vaccine:

Date administered:

Next Dose date:

Administered by:

Vaccine:

Date administered:

Next Dose date:

Administered by:

Vaccine:

Date administered:

Next Dose date:

Administered by:

Vaccine:

Date administered:

Next Dose date:

Administered by:

Vaccine:

Date administered:

Next Dose date:

Administered by:

Vaccine:

Date administered:

Next Dose date:

Administered by:

Vaccine:

Date administered:

Next Dose date:

Administered by:

IMMUNIZATION RECORD

Vaccine:

Date administered:

Next Dose date:

Administered by:

Vaccine:

Date administered:

Next Dose date:

Administered by:

Vaccine:

Date administered:

Next Dose date:

Administered by:

Vaccine:

Date administered:

Next Dose date:

Administered by:

Vaccine:

Date administered:

Next Dose date:

Administered by:

Vaccine:

Date administered:

Next Dose date:

Administered by:

Vaccine:

Date administered:

Next Dose date:

Administered by:

Vaccine:

Date administered:

Next Dose date:

Administered by:

Vaccine:

Date administered:

Next Dose date:

Administered by:

Vaccine:

Date administered:

Next Dose date:

Administered by:

Vaccine:

Date administered:

Next Dose date:

Administered by:

Vaccine:

Date administered:

Next Dose date:

Administered by:

IMMUNIZATION RECORD

Vaccine:

Date administered:

Next Dose date:

Administered by:

Vaccine:

Date administered:

Next Dose date:

Administered by:

Vaccine:

Date administered:

Next Dose date:

Administered by:

Vaccine:

Date administered:

Next Dose date:

Administered by:

Vaccine:

Date administered:

Next Dose date:

Administered by:

Vaccine:

Date administered:

Next Dose date:

Administered by:

Vaccine:

Date administered:

Next Dose date:

Administered by:

Vaccine:

Date administered:

Next Dose date:

Administered by:

Vaccine:

Date administered:

Next Dose date:

Administered by:

Vaccine:

Date administered:

Next Dose date:

Administered by:

Vaccine:

Date administered:

Next Dose date:

Administered by:

Vaccine:

Date administered:

Next Dose date:

Administered by:

IMMUNIZATION RECORD

Vaccine:

Date administered:

Next Dose date:

Administered by:

Vaccine:

Date administered:

Next Dose date:

Administered by:

Vaccine:

Date administered:

Next Dose date:

Administered by:

Vaccine:

Date administered:

Next Dose date:

Administered by:

Vaccine:

Date administered:

Next Dose date:

Administered by:

Vaccine:

Date administered:

Next Dose date:

Administered by:

Vaccine:

Date administered:

Next Dose date:

Administered by:

Vaccine:

Date administered:

Next Dose date:

Administered by:

Vaccine:

Date administered:

Next Dose date:

Administered by:

Vaccine:

Date administered:

Next Dose date:

Administered by:

Vaccine:

Date administered:

Next Dose date:

Administered by:

Vaccine:

Date administered:

Next Dose date:

Administered by:

TREATMENT HISTORY- MEDICATION

MEDICATION NAME	DATE STARTED	START DOSE	DATE ENDED	END DOSE
FREQUENCY				
PRESCRIBING PHYSICIAN				
RESULT & NOTES				

MEDICATION NAME	DATE STARTED	START DOSE	DATE ENDED	END DOSE
FREQUENCY				
PRESCRIBING PHYSICIAN				
RESULT & NOTES				

MEDICATION NAME	DATE STARTED	START DOSE	DATE ENDED	END DOSE
FREQUENCY				
PRESCRIBING PHYSICIAN				
RESULT & NOTES				

TREATMENT HISTORY- MEDICATION

MEDICATION NAME	DATE STARTED	START DOSE	DATE ENDED	END DOSE
FREQUENCY				
PRESCRIBING PHYSICIAN				
RESULT & NOTES				

MEDICATION NAME	DATE STARTED	START DOSE	DATE ENDED	END DOSE
FREQUENCY				
PRESCRIBING PHYSICIAN				
RESULT & NOTES				

MEDICATION NAME	DATE STARTED	START DOSE	DATE ENDED	END DOSE
FREQUENCY				
PRESCRIBING PHYSICIAN				
RESULT & NOTES				

TREATMENT HISTORY- MEDICATION

MEDICATION NAME	DATE STARTED	START DOSE	DATE ENDED	END DOSE
FREQUENCY				
PRESCRIBING PHYSICIAN				
RESULT & NOTES				

MEDICATION NAME	DATE STARTED	START DOSE	DATE ENDED	END DOSE
FREQUENCY				
PRESCRIBING PHYSICIAN				
RESULT & NOTES				

MEDICATION NAME	DATE STARTED	START DOSE	DATE ENDED	END DOSE
FREQUENCY				
PRESCRIBING PHYSICIAN				
RESULT & NOTES				

TREATMENT HISTORY- MEDICATION

MEDICATION NAME	DATE STARTED	START DOSE	DATE ENDED	END DOSE
FREQUENCY				
PRESCRIBING PHYSICIAN				
RESULT & NOTES				

MEDICATION NAME	DATE STARTED	START DOSE	DATE ENDED	END DOSE
FREQUENCY				
PRESCRIBING PHYSICIAN				
RESULT & NOTES				

MEDICATION NAME	DATE STARTED	START DOSE	DATE ENDED	END DOSE
FREQUENCY				
PRESCRIBING PHYSICIAN				
RESULT & NOTES				

TREATMENT HISTORY- MEDICATION

MEDICATION NAME	DATE STARTED	START DOSE	DATE ENDED	END DOSE

FREQUENCY	
PRESCRIBING PHYSICIAN	
RESULT & NOTES	

MEDICATION NAME	DATE STARTED	START DOSE	DATE ENDED	END DOSE

FREQUENCY	
PRESCRIBING PHYSICIAN	
RESULT & NOTES	

MEDICATION NAME	DATE STARTED	START DOSE	DATE ENDED	END DOSE

FREQUENCY	
PRESCRIBING PHYSICIAN	
RESULT & NOTES	

TREATMENT HISTORY- MEDICATION

MEDICATION NAME	DATE STARTED	START DOSE	DATE ENDED	END DOSE
FREQUENCY				
PRESCRIBING PHYSICIAN				
RESULT & NOTES				

MEDICATION NAME	DATE STARTED	START DOSE	DATE ENDED	END DOSE
FREQUENCY				
PRESCRIBING PHYSICIAN				
RESULT & NOTES				

MEDICATION NAME	DATE STARTED	START DOSE	DATE ENDED	END DOSE
FREQUENCY				
PRESCRIBING PHYSICIAN				
RESULT & NOTES				

TREATMENT HISTORY- MEDICATION

MEDICATION NAME	DATE STARTED	START DOSE	DATE ENDED	END DOSE

FREQUENCY	
PRESCRIBING PHYSICIAN	
RESULT & NOTES	

MEDICATION NAME	DATE STARTED	START DOSE	DATE ENDED	END DOSE

FREQUENCY	
PRESCRIBING PHYSICIAN	
RESULT & NOTES	

MEDICATION NAME	DATE STARTED	START DOSE	DATE ENDED	END DOSE

FREQUENCY	
PRESCRIBING PHYSICIAN	
RESULT & NOTES	

TREATMENT HISTORY- MEDICATION

MEDICATION NAME	DATE STARTED	START DOSE	DATE ENDED	END DOSE
FREQUENCY				
PRESCRIBING PHYSICIAN				
RESULT & NOTES				

MEDICATION NAME	DATE STARTED	START DOSE	DATE ENDED	END DOSE
FREQUENCY				
PRESCRIBING PHYSICIAN				
RESULT & NOTES				

MEDICATION NAME	DATE STARTED	START DOSE	DATE ENDED	END DOSE
FREQUENCY				
PRESCRIBING PHYSICIAN				
RESULT & NOTES				

TREATMENT HISTORY- MEDICATION

MEDICATION NAME	DATE STARTED	START DOSE	DATE ENDED	END DOSE

FREQUENCY	
PRESCRIBING PHYSICIAN	
RESULT & NOTES	

MEDICATION NAME	DATE STARTED	START DOSE	DATE ENDED	END DOSE

FREQUENCY	
PRESCRIBING PHYSICIAN	
RESULT & NOTES	

MEDICATION NAME	DATE STARTED	START DOSE	DATE ENDED	END DOSE

FREQUENCY	
PRESCRIBING PHYSICIAN	
RESULT & NOTES	

TREATMENT HISTORY- MEDICATION

MEDICATION NAME	DATE STARTED	START DOSE	DATE ENDED	END DOSE
FREQUENCY				
PRESCRIBING PHYSICIAN				
RESULT & NOTES				

MEDICATION NAME	DATE STARTED	START DOSE	DATE ENDED	END DOSE
FREQUENCY				
PRESCRIBING PHYSICIAN				
RESULT & NOTES				

MEDICATION NAME	DATE STARTED	START DOSE	DATE ENDED	END DOSE
FREQUENCY				
PRESCRIBING PHYSICIAN				
RESULT & NOTES				

TREATMENT HISTORY- MEDICATION

MEDICATION NAME	DATE STARTED	START DOSE	DATE ENDED	END DOSE

FREQUENCY	
PRESCRIBING PHYSICIAN	
RESULT & NOTES	

MEDICATION NAME	DATE STARTED	START DOSE	DATE ENDED	END DOSE

FREQUENCY	
PRESCRIBING PHYSICIAN	
RESULT & NOTES	

MEDICATION NAME	DATE STARTED	START DOSE	DATE ENDED	END DOSE

FREQUENCY	
PRESCRIBING PHYSICIAN	
RESULT & NOTES	

TREATMENT HISTORY- MEDICATION

MEDICATION NAME	DATE STARTED	START DOSE	DATE ENDED	END DOSE

FREQUENCY	
PRESCRIBING PHYSICIAN	
RESULT & NOTES	

MEDICATION NAME	DATE STARTED	START DOSE	DATE ENDED	END DOSE

FREQUENCY	
PRESCRIBING PHYSICIAN	
RESULT & NOTES	

MEDICATION NAME	DATE STARTED	START DOSE	DATE ENDED	END DOSE

FREQUENCY	
PRESCRIBING PHYSICIAN	
RESULT & NOTES	

SYMPTOM TRACKER

DATE & TIME	
DESCRIPTION	
BODY TEMPERATURE	
OBSERVATIONS	

PHYSICAL SYMPTOMS	FEVER		SNEEZING		RASH		Other	
POSSIBLE TRIGGERS	FOOD		WEATHER		MEDICATION		Other	

ACTION TAKEN	

DATE & TIME	
DESCRIPTION	
BODY TEMPERATURE	
OBSERVATIONS	

PHYSICAL SYMPTOMS	FEVER		SNEEZING		RASH		Other	
POSSIBLE TRIGGERS	FOOD		WEATHER		MEDICATION		Other	

ACTION TAKEN	

DATE & TIME	
DESCRIPTION	

BODY TEMPERATURE	
OBSERVATIONS	

PHYSICAL SYMPTOMS	FEVER		SNEEZING		RASH		Other	
POSSIBLE TRIGGERS	FOOD		WEATHER		MEDICATION		Other	

ACTION TAKEN	

DATE & TIME	
DESCRIPTION	

BODY TEMPERATURE	
OBSERVATIONS	

PHYSICAL SYMPTOMS	FEVER		SNEEZING		RASH		Other	
POSSIBLE TRIGGERS	FOOD		WEATHER		MEDICATION		Other	

ACTION TAKEN	

SYMPTOM TRACKER

DATE & TIME	
DESCRIPTION	
BODY TEMPERATURE	
OBSERVATIONS	

PHYSICAL SYMPTOMS	FEVER		SNEEZING		RASH		Other	
POSSIBLE TRIGGERS	FOOD		WEATHER		MEDICATION		Other	

ACTION TAKEN	

DATE & TIME	
DESCRIPTION	
BODY TEMPERATURE	
OBSERVATIONS	

PHYSICAL SYMPTOMS	FEVER		SNEEZING		RASH		Other	
POSSIBLE TRIGGERS	FOOD		WEATHER		MEDICATION		Other	

ACTION TAKEN	

SYMPTOM TRACKER

DATE & TIME	
DESCRIPTION	
BODY TEMPERATURE	
OBSERVATIONS	

PHYSICAL SYMPTOMS	FEVER		SNEEZING		RASH		Other	
POSSIBLE TRIGGERS	FOOD		WEATHER		MEDICATION		Other	

ACTION TAKEN	

DATE & TIME	
DESCRIPTION	
BODY TEMPERATURE	
OBSERVATIONS	

PHYSICAL SYMPTOMS	FEVER		SNEEZING		RASH		Other	
POSSIBLE TRIGGERS	FOOD		WEATHER		MEDICATION		Other	

ACTION TAKEN	

SYMPTOM TRACKER

DATE & TIME	
DESCRIPTION	
BODY TEMPERATURE	
OBSERVATIONS	

PHYSICAL SYMPTOMS	FEVER		SNEEZING		RASH		Other	
POSSIBLE TRIGGERS	FOOD		WEATHER		MEDICATION		Other	

ACTION TAKEN	

DATE & TIME	
DESCRIPTION	
BODY TEMPERATURE	
OBSERVATIONS	

PHYSICAL SYMPTOMS	FEVER		SNEEZING		RASH		Other	
POSSIBLE TRIGGERS	FOOD		WEATHER		MEDICATION		Other	

ACTION TAKEN	

SYMPTOM TRACKER

DATE & TIME	
DESCRIPTION	
BODY TEMPERATURE	
OBSERVATIONS	

PHYSICAL SYMPTOMS	FEVER		SNEEZING		RASH		Other	
POSSIBLE TRIGGERS	FOOD		WEATHER		MEDICATION		Other	

ACTION TAKEN	

DATE & TIME	
DESCRIPTION	
BODY TEMPERATURE	
OBSERVATIONS	

PHYSICAL SYMPTOMS	FEVER		SNEEZING		RASH		Other	
POSSIBLE TRIGGERS	FOOD		WEATHER		MEDICATION		Other	

ACTION TAKEN	

SYMPTOM TRACKER

DATE & TIME	
DESCRIPTION	
BODY TEMPERATURE	
OBSERVATIONS	

PHYSICAL SYMPTOMS	FEVER		SNEEZING		RASH		Other	
POSSIBLE TRIGGERS	FOOD		WEATHER		MEDICATION		Other	

ACTION TAKEN	

DATE & TIME	
DESCRIPTION	
BODY TEMPERATURE	
OBSERVATIONS	

PHYSICAL SYMPTOMS	FEVER		SNEEZING		RASH		Other	
POSSIBLE TRIGGERS	FOOD		WEATHER		MEDICATION		Other	

ACTION TAKEN	

SYMPTOM TRACKER

DATE & TIME	
DESCRIPTION	
BODY TEMPERATURE	
OBSERVATIONS	

PHYSICAL SYMPTOMS	FEVER		SNEEZING		RASH		Other	
POSSIBLE TRIGGERS	FOOD		WEATHER		MEDICATION		Other	

ACTION TAKEN

DATE & TIME	
DESCRIPTION	
BODY TEMPERATURE	
OBSERVATIONS	

PHYSICAL SYMPTOMS	FEVER		SNEEZING		RASH		Other	
POSSIBLE TRIGGERS	FOOD		WEATHER		MEDICATION		Other	

ACTION TAKEN

SYMPTOM TRACKER

DATE & TIME	
DESCRIPTION	
BODY TEMPERATURE	
OBSERVATIONS	

PHYSICAL SYMPTOMS	FEVER		SNEEZING		RASH		Other	
POSSIBLE TRIGGERS	FOOD		WEATHER		MEDICATION		Other	

ACTION TAKEN	

DATE & TIME	
DESCRIPTION	
BODY TEMPERATURE	
OBSERVATIONS	

PHYSICAL SYMPTOMS	FEVER		SNEEZING		RASH		Other	
POSSIBLE TRIGGERS	FOOD		WEATHER		MEDICATION		Other	

ACTION TAKEN	

SYMPTOM TRACKER

DATE & TIME	
DESCRIPTION	
BODY TEMPERATURE	
OBSERVATIONS	

PHYSICAL SYMPTOMS	FEVER		SNEEZING		RASH		Other	
POSSIBLE TRIGGERS	FOOD		WEATHER		MEDICATION		Other	

ACTION TAKEN	

DATE & TIME	
DESCRIPTION	
BODY TEMPERATURE	
OBSERVATIONS	

PHYSICAL SYMPTOMS	FEVER		SNEEZING		RASH		Other	
POSSIBLE TRIGGERS	FOOD		WEATHER		MEDICATION		Other	

ACTION TAKEN	

SYMPTOM TRACKER

DATE & TIME	
DESCRIPTION	
BODY TEMPERATURE	
OBSERVATIONS	

PHYSICAL SYMPTOMS	FEVER		SNEEZING		RASH		Other	
POSSIBLE TRIGGERS	FOOD		WEATHER		MEDICATION		Other	

ACTION TAKEN	

DATE & TIME	
DESCRIPTION	
BODY TEMPERATURE	
OBSERVATIONS	

PHYSICAL SYMPTOMS	FEVER		SNEEZING		RASH		Other	
POSSIBLE TRIGGERS	FOOD		WEATHER		MEDICATION		Other	

ACTION TAKEN	

DATE & TIME	
DESCRIPTION	

BODY TEMPERATURE	
OBSERVATIONS	

PHYSICAL SYMPTOMS	FEVER		SNEEZING		RASH		Other	
POSSIBLE TRIGGERS	FOOD		WEATHER		MEDICATION		Other	

ACTION TAKEN	

DATE & TIME	
DESCRIPTION	

BODY TEMPERATURE	
OBSERVATIONS	

PHYSICAL SYMPTOMS	FEVER		SNEEZING		RASH		Other	
POSSIBLE TRIGGERS	FOOD		WEATHER		MEDICATION		Other	

ACTION TAKEN	

SYMPTOM TRACKER

DATE & TIME	
DESCRIPTION	
BODY TEMPERATURE	
OBSERVATIONS	

PHYSICAL SYMPTOMS	FEVER		SNEEZING		RASH		Other	
POSSIBLE TRIGGERS	FOOD		WEATHER		MEDICATION		Other	
ACTION TAKEN								

DATE & TIME	
DESCRIPTION	
BODY TEMPERATURE	
OBSERVATIONS	

PHYSICAL SYMPTOMS	FEVER		SNEEZING		RASH		Other	
POSSIBLE TRIGGERS	FOOD		WEATHER		MEDICATION		Other	
ACTION TAKEN								

DATE & TIME	
DESCRIPTION	

BODY TEMPERATURE	
OBSERVATIONS	

PHYSICAL SYMPTOMS	FEVER		SNEEZING		RASH		Other	
POSSIBLE TRIGGERS	FOOD		WEATHER		MEDICATION		Other	
ACTION TAKEN								

DATE & TIME	
DESCRIPTION	

BODY TEMPERATURE	
OBSERVATIONS	

PHYSICAL SYMPTOMS	FEVER		SNEEZING		RASH		Other	
POSSIBLE TRIGGERS	FOOD		WEATHER		MEDICATION		Other	
ACTION TAKEN								

SYMPTOM TRACKER

DATE & TIME	
DESCRIPTION	
BODY TEMPERATURE	
OBSERVATIONS	

PHYSICAL SYMPTOMS	FEVER		SNEEZING		RASH		Other	
POSSIBLE TRIGGERS	FOOD		WEATHER		MEDICATION		Other	

ACTION TAKEN	

DATE & TIME	
DESCRIPTION	
BODY TEMPERATURE	
OBSERVATIONS	

PHYSICAL SYMPTOMS	FEVER		SNEEZING		RASH		Other	
POSSIBLE TRIGGERS	FOOD		WEATHER		MEDICATION		Other	

ACTION TAKEN	

DATE & TIME	
DESCRIPTION	
BODY TEMPERATURE	
OBSERVATIONS	

PHYSICAL SYMPTOMS	FEVER		SNEEZING		RASH		Other	
POSSIBLE TRIGGERS	FOOD		WEATHER		MEDICATION		Other	

ACTION TAKEN	

DATE & TIME	
DESCRIPTION	
BODY TEMPERATURE	
OBSERVATIONS	

PHYSICAL SYMPTOMS	FEVER		SNEEZING		RASH		Other	
POSSIBLE TRIGGERS	FOOD		WEATHER		MEDICATION		Other	

ACTION TAKEN	

SYMPTOM TRACKER

DATE & TIME	
DESCRIPTION	
BODY TEMPERATURE	
OBSERVATIONS	

PHYSICAL SYMPTOMS	FEVER		SNEEZING		RASH		Other	
POSSIBLE TRIGGERS	FOOD		WEATHER		MEDICATION		Other	

ACTION TAKEN	

DATE & TIME	
DESCRIPTION	
BODY TEMPERATURE	
OBSERVATIONS	

PHYSICAL SYMPTOMS	FEVER		SNEEZING		RASH		Other	
POSSIBLE TRIGGERS	FOOD		WEATHER		MEDICATION		Other	

ACTION TAKEN	

SYMPTOM TRACKER

DATE & TIME	
DESCRIPTION	

BODY TEMPERATURE	
OBSERVATIONS	

PHYSICAL SYMPTOMS	FEVER		SNEEZING		RASH		Other	
POSSIBLE TRIGGERS	FOOD		WEATHER		MEDICATION		Other	

ACTION TAKEN	

DATE & TIME	
DESCRIPTION	

BODY TEMPERATURE	
OBSERVATIONS	

PHYSICAL SYMPTOMS	FEVER		SNEEZING		RASH		Other	
POSSIBLE TRIGGERS	FOOD		WEATHER		MEDICATION		Other	

ACTION TAKEN	

SYMPTOM TRACKER

DATE & TIME	
DESCRIPTION	

BODY TEMPERATURE

OBSERVATIONS	

PHYSICAL SYMPTOMS	FEVER		SNEEZING		RASH		Other	
POSSIBLE TRIGGERS	FOOD		WEATHER		MEDICATION		Other	

ACTION TAKEN

DATE & TIME	
DESCRIPTION	

BODY TEMPERATURE

OBSERVATIONS	

PHYSICAL SYMPTOMS	FEVER		SNEEZING		RASH		Other	
POSSIBLE TRIGGERS	FOOD		WEATHER		MEDICATION		Other	

ACTION TAKEN

DATE & TIME	
DESCRIPTION	
BODY TEMPERATURE	
OBSERVATIONS	

PHYSICAL SYMPTOMS	FEVER		SNEEZING		RASH		Other	
POSSIBLE TRIGGERS	FOOD		WEATHER		MEDICATION		Other	

ACTION TAKEN	

DATE & TIME	
DESCRIPTION	
BODY TEMPERATURE	
OBSERVATIONS	

PHYSICAL SYMPTOMS	FEVER		SNEEZING		RASH		Other	
POSSIBLE TRIGGERS	FOOD		WEATHER		MEDICATION		Other	

ACTION TAKEN	

TREATMENT HISTORY- VISITS

DATE	TIME	LOCATION

REASON FOR VISIT	

TEST	
RESULT	
DIAGNOSIS	
TREATMENT	
NOTES	

DATE	TIME	LOCATION

REASON FOR VISIT	

TEST	
RESULT	
DIAGNOSIS	
TREATMENT	
NOTES	

DATE	TIME	LOCATION

REASON FOR VISIT	

	TEST	
	RESULT	
	DIAGNOSIS	
	TREATMENT	
	NOTES	

DATE	TIME	LOCATION

REASON FOR VISIT	

	TEST	
	RESULT	
	DIAGNOSIS	
	TREATMENT	
	NOTES	

TREATMENT HISTORY- VISITS

DATE	TIME	LOCATION

REASON FOR VISIT	

TEST	
RESULT	
DIAGNOSIS	
TREATMENT	
NOTES	

DATE	TIME	LOCATION

REASON FOR VISIT	

TEST	
RESULT	
DIAGNOSIS	
TREATMENT	
NOTES	

TREATMENT HISTORY- VISITS

DATE	TIME	LOCATION
REASON FOR VISIT		

TEST	
RESULT	
DIAGNOSIS	
TREATMENT	
NOTES	

DATE	TIME	LOCATION
REASON FOR VISIT		

TEST	
RESULT	
DIAGNOSIS	
TREATMENT	
NOTES	

TREATMENT HISTORY- VISITS

DATE	TIME	LOCATION

REASON FOR VISIT	

TEST	
RESULT	
DIAGNOSIS	
TREATMENT	
NOTES	

DATE	TIME	LOCATION

REASON FOR VISIT	

TEST	
RESULT	
DIAGNOSIS	
TREATMENT	
NOTES	

DATE	TIME	LOCATION

REASON FOR VISIT	

TEST	
RESULT	
DIAGNOSIS	
TREATMENT	
NOTES	

DATE	TIME	LOCATION

REASON FOR VISIT	

TEST	
RESULT	
DIAGNOSIS	
TREATMENT	
NOTES	

TREATMENT HISTORY- VISITS

DATE	TIME	LOCATION

REASON FOR VISIT	

TEST	
RESULT	
DIAGNOSIS	
TREATMENT	
NOTES	

DATE	TIME	LOCATION

REASON FOR VISIT	

TEST	
RESULT	
DIAGNOSIS	
TREATMENT	
NOTES	

DATE	TIME	LOCATION

REASON FOR VISIT	

TEST	
RESULT	
DIAGNOSIS	
TREATMENT	
NOTES	

DATE	TIME	LOCATION

REASON FOR VISIT	

TEST	
RESULT	
DIAGNOSIS	
TREATMENT	
NOTES	

TREATMENT HISTORY- VISITS

DATE	TIME	LOCATION

REASON FOR VISIT	

TEST	
RESULT	
DIAGNOSIS	
TREATMENT	
NOTES	

DATE	TIME	LOCATION

REASON FOR VISIT	

TEST	
RESULT	
DIAGNOSIS	
TREATMENT	
NOTES	

TREATMENT HISTORY- VISITS

DATE	TIME	LOCATION
REASON FOR VISIT		

TEST		
RESULT		
DIAGNOSIS		
TREATMENT		
NOTES		

DATE	TIME	LOCATION
REASON FOR VISIT		

TEST		
RESULT		
DIAGNOSIS		
TREATMENT		
NOTES		

TREATMENT HISTORY- VISITS

DATE	TIME	LOCATION

REASON FOR VISIT	

TEST	
RESULT	
DIAGNOSIS	
TREATMENT	
NOTES	

DATE	TIME	LOCATION

REASON FOR VISIT	

TEST	
RESULT	
DIAGNOSIS	
TREATMENT	
NOTES	

TREATMENT HISTORY- VISITS

DATE	TIME	LOCATION
REASON FOR VISIT		

TEST	
RESULT	
DIAGNOSIS	
TREATMENT	
NOTES	

DATE	TIME	LOCATION
REASON FOR VISIT		

TEST	
RESULT	
DIAGNOSIS	
TREATMENT	
NOTES	

TREATMENT HISTORY- VISITS

DATE	TIME	LOCATION

REASON FOR VISIT	

TEST	
RESULT	
DIAGNOSIS	
TREATMENT	
NOTES	

DATE	TIME	LOCATION

REASON FOR VISIT	

TEST	
RESULT	
DIAGNOSIS	
TREATMENT	
NOTES	

DATE	TIME	LOCATION

REASON FOR VISIT	

TEST	
RESULT	
DIAGNOSIS	
TREATMENT	
NOTES	

DATE	TIME	LOCATION

REASON FOR VISIT	

TEST	
RESULT	
DIAGNOSIS	
TREATMENT	
NOTES	

TREATMENT HISTORY- VISITS

DATE	TIME	LOCATION

REASON FOR VISIT	

TEST	
RESULT	
DIAGNOSIS	
TREATMENT	
NOTES	

DATE	TIME	LOCATION

REASON FOR VISIT	

TEST	
RESULT	
DIAGNOSIS	
TREATMENT	
NOTES	

DATE	TIME	LOCATION
REASON FOR VISIT		

TEST	
RESULT	
DIAGNOSIS	
TREATMENT	
NOTES	

DATE	TIME	LOCATION
REASON FOR VISIT		

TEST	
RESULT	
DIAGNOSIS	
TREATMENT	
NOTES	

TREATMENT HISTORY- VISITS

DATE	TIME	LOCATION

REASON FOR VISIT	

TEST	
RESULT	
DIAGNOSIS	
TREATMENT	
NOTES	

DATE	TIME	LOCATION

REASON FOR VISIT	

TEST	
RESULT	
DIAGNOSIS	
TREATMENT	
NOTES	

TREATMENT HISTORY- VISITS

DATE	TIME	LOCATION

REASON FOR VISIT	

	TEST	
	RESULT	
	DIAGNOSIS	
	TREATMENT	
	NOTES	

DATE	TIME	LOCATION

REASON FOR VISIT	

	TEST	
	RESULT	
	DIAGNOSIS	
	TREATMENT	
	NOTES	

TREATMENT HISTORY- VISITS

DATE	TIME	LOCATION

REASON FOR VISIT	

TEST	
RESULT	
DIAGNOSIS	
TREATMENT	
NOTES	

DATE	TIME	LOCATION

REASON FOR VISIT	

TEST	
RESULT	
DIAGNOSIS	
TREATMENT	
NOTES	

TREATMENT HISTORY- VISITS

DATE	TIME	LOCATION

REASON FOR VISIT	

TEST	
RESULT	
DIAGNOSIS	
TREATMENT	
NOTES	

DATE	TIME	LOCATION

REASON FOR VISIT	

TEST	
RESULT	
DIAGNOSIS	
TREATMENT	
NOTES	

TREATMENT HISTORY- VISITS

DATE	TIME	LOCATION

REASON FOR VISIT	

TEST	
RESULT	
DIAGNOSIS	
TREATMENT	
NOTES	

DATE	TIME	LOCATION

REASON FOR VISIT	

TEST	
RESULT	
DIAGNOSIS	
TREATMENT	
NOTES	

TREATMENT HISTORY- VISITS

DATE	TIME	LOCATION

REASON FOR VISIT	

TEST	
RESULT	
DIAGNOSIS	
TREATMENT	
NOTES	

DATE	TIME	LOCATION

REASON FOR VISIT	

TEST	
RESULT	
DIAGNOSIS	
TREATMENT	
NOTES	

TREATMENT HISTORY- VISITS

DATE	TIME	LOCATION

REASON FOR VISIT	

TEST	
RESULT	
DIAGNOSIS	
TREATMENT	
NOTES	

DATE	TIME	LOCATION

REASON FOR VISIT	

TEST	
RESULT	
DIAGNOSIS	
TREATMENT	
NOTES	

DATE	TIME	LOCATION

REASON FOR VISIT	

TEST	
RESULT	
DIAGNOSIS	
TREATMENT	
NOTES	

DATE	TIME	LOCATION

REASON FOR VISIT	

TEST	
RESULT	
DIAGNOSIS	
TREATMENT	
NOTES	

GROWTH LOG

DATE	AGE	HEIGHT

WEIGHT LOG

DATE	AGE	WEIGHT

GROWTH LOG

DATE	AGE	HEIGHT

WEIGHT LOG

DATE	AGE	WEIGHT

TOOTH CHART

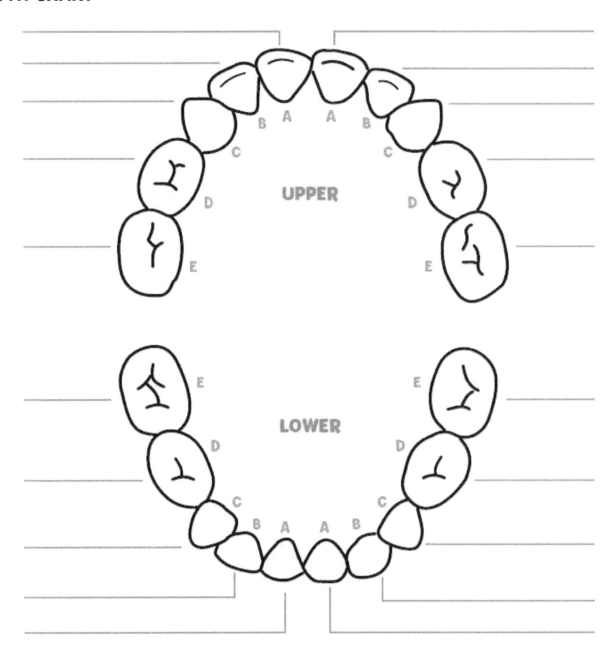

UPPER

LOWER

A. Central Incisor   B. Lateral Incisor   C. Cuspid   D. First Molar   E. Second Molar

TOOTH RECORD- ADULT TEETH

TOOTH LOCATION	DATE

NOTES

NOTES

NOTES

NOTES

NOTES

NOTES

NOTES

NOTES

Made in the USA
Monee, IL
29 June 2022

98821404R00052